Eduardo Barbosa Ferreira

SBAV in paediatrics

Eduardo Barbosa Ferreira

SBAV in paediatrics

An analysis of theoretical knowledge

ScienciaScripts

Imprint

Cover image: www.ingimage.com

This book is a translation from the original published under ISBN 978-613-9-71801-6.

Publisher:
Sciencia Scripts
is a trademark of
Dodo Books Indian Ocean Ltd. and OmniScriptum S.R.L publishing group

120 High Road, East Finchley, London, N2 9ED, United Kingdom
Str. Armeneasca 28/1, office 1, Chisinau MD-2012, Republic of Moldova, Europe
Printed at: see last page
ISBN: 978-620-7-95900-6

SUMMARY

Nurses' role in basic and advanced life support in paediatrics: an analysis of theoretical knowledge[1]

Eduardo Ferreira[2] , Marislei Espíndula Brasileiro[3 4] ,

Summary

The aim of this study was to carry out a literature review to analyse the role of nurses and the importance of their theoretical and scientific knowledge in basic and advanced life support in paediatrics. Materials and Methods: This was a descriptive, exploratory study, with an integrative analysis of the literature available in virtual databases. This study identified an insufficient number of studies on the subject under investigation. It was possible to conclude that the nursing team's knowledge on this subject is still incipient. This study made it possible to identify the importance of nurses' theoretical and scientific knowledge within institutions that care for children at risk of cardiac arrest. This knowledge enables them to provide more agile care by organising the team based on their theoretical background. Therefore, there is a need to invest in training for professionals who provide direct assistance to patients in cardiac arrest.

Keywords: advanced life support, basic life support, cardiac arrest, child, paediatrics.

---

[1] Article presented to the Postgraduate Course in Nursing.., class no. ...., at the Centre for Nursing .... Studies.
Nursing and Nutrition Studies/Pontifical Catholic University of Goiás.

[2] Nurse, specialising in .... , e-mail:..., ... ,.....
[3] PhD in Health Sciences - FM-UFG, PhD - PUC-Go, Master's in Nursing - UFMG, Nurse, Professor at CEEN, e-mail: marislei@cultura.trd.br
[4] Nurse......................

CHAPTER 1

Introduction

The interest or motivation to research the role of nurses in basic and advanced life support in paediatrics arose from the observation that the preparation and theoretical knowledge of nurses in Basic Life Support (BLS) and Advanced Life Support (ALS) is of paramount importance for successful cardiopulmonary resuscitation and that there are still few scientific studies focusing on children. This is probably because theoretical knowledge supports the work of nurses (ALVES, BARBOSA, FARIA, 2013).

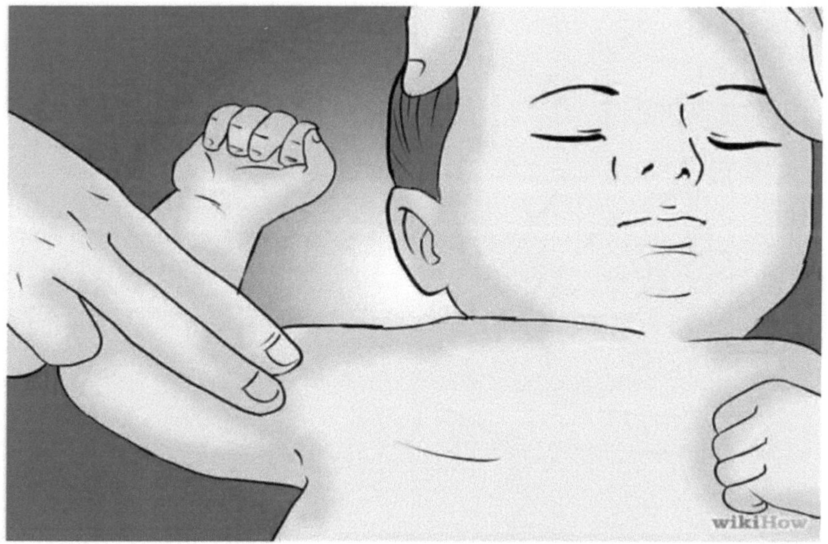

VNS is the first care the victim receives and includes airway clearance, ventilation and artificial circulation (FERREIRA, 2001). The main characteristic of VNS in Brazil is that no invasive manoeuvres are performed on the patient, which is why it can be carried out by untrained personnel, but remote medical assistance is of the utmost importance. VAS, on the other hand, can only be carried out by trained professionals, such as doctors and nurses, and therefore allows invasive procedures, such as respiratory access with a definitive airway and venous access with volume replacement and administration of medication (BRASIL, 2002).

BLS or VAS teams are often called in to deal with paediatric emergencies. Paediatrics is a speciality that deals with children's problems in two main ways: the first is childcare, which deals with prevention and maintaining normal conditions, and the other is clinical paediatrics, also known as curative paediatrics, which deals with restoring the child's health when it is altered (GUSSON E LOPES, 2010).

World and national rates of death due to CA or cardiovascular disease.

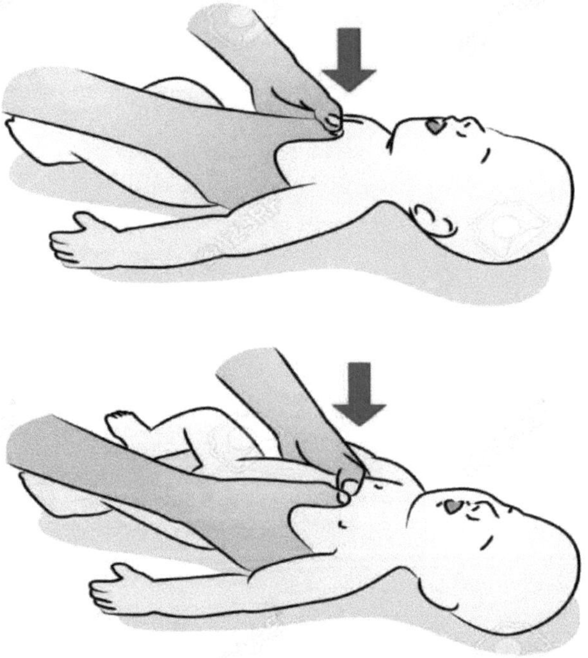

One of the most serious situations in paediatrics that puts a child's life at risk is cardiac arrest. The definition of CA is given as the interruption of mechanical and respiratory activity, the diagnosis is made based on the observation of the absence of a pulse in the great arteries, which is configured as circulatory arrest (MATSUMO, 2012).

One of the most important determinants of success in cardiopulmonary resuscitation (CPR) is the theoretical knowledge and practical skills of the BLS and VAS teams. The teams that carry out BLS and VAS manoeuvres need to be well-trained teams, because quick and effective action in the face of cardiopulmonary arrest means a greater chance of patient recovery. In this sense, nursing professionals are of the utmost importance, as they are usually the first to witness a cardiac arrest in hospital, and are the ones who most often call the response team. These professionals therefore need to have up-to-date technical knowledge and developed practical skills in order to contribute more effectively to CPR manoeuvres. The chance of survival after a cardiac arrest varies from two to 49 per cent, depending on the initial heart rhythm and the early start of resuscitation (FILGUEIRAS-FILHO et al., 2006; GOMBOTZ et al., 2006; MOULE and ALBARRAN, 2002; HORSTED et al., 2007).

In this context, the nurse's role is of paramount importance in the event of CPR, since the occurrence is unexpected and requires the nursing team to identify and recognise the patient in this situation, master the previous diagnosis, and have the skills and training to provide effective care. This is why the professional training offered to team members who work specifically in the emergency department needs to be more effective in order to provide them with up-to-date knowledge and develop their skills in assisting patients with CPR, whether they are children or adults (ARAÚJO et. al, 2012).

Various factors put children at risk. Among the causes that require assistance in paediatric care units are respiratory diseases, convulsive states, poisoning, accidents and traumas, often leading to cardiorespiratory arrest, which is the most important medical emergency in paediatrics. Infectious, parasitic and traumatic processes are often the main causes of admission to these units (TACSI; VENDRUSCOLO, 2004).

In order to make sense of this work, it is important to define Cardio-Respiratory Arrest (CRA). CA is defined as the cessation of clinically detectable cardiac mechanical activity. It is characterised by unresponsiveness, apnoea and the absence of a detectable central pulse. In infants and children, most CA results in progressive respiratory failure or shock, or both. Less commonly, they can occur without warning or secondary to an arrhythmia (AHA, 2008).

From the 1960s onwards, VAS and CPR care developed through standardised programmes and procedures, resulting from proposals from international organisations for emergency training. In the 1980s, paediatric and neonatal CPR care was standardised as Paediatric BLS and VAS. These training courses in paediatric CPR were introduced in Brazil in 1998 by the Brazilian Society of Cardiology, in agreement with the Brazilian Society of Cardiology.

Brazilian Society of Paediatrics, prioritising the training of medical professionals and, subsequently, nursing professionals (ALMEIDA et al, 2011).

When children are in the acute phase of illness or accidents, they arrive at emergency services with a high risk of death, requiring the care team to develop its potential to provide emergency care. The nursing team is responsible for the intensive care of critically ill patients, through permanent assessment, vigilance and carrying out procedures and techniques that complement medical therapy. They must also have protocols for nursing care, guaranteeing the continuity of an integrated approach with the medical team, providing guidance and welcoming family members. BLS is very important, as only 1/3 of children who suffer cardiac arrest receive BLS. This is why CPR manoeuvres should be taught to the whole of society, since it has been shown that out-of-hospital respiratory arrest care by lay rescuers can have the greatest impact on survival without neurological sequelae (TACSII; VENDRUSCOLO, 2004).

Lima et. al, (2009) found a significant impact on the level of knowledge of nursing professionals after training in BLS and VAS, as can be seen by the 91 per cent gain in knowledge in the total sample, reaching 131 per cent in the group of nursing assistants. These data corroborate the need to structure continuing health education as a tool that will help improve CPR success rates.

In general, when compared to adults, pre-hospital primary cardiac arrest is a less frequent etiology of CA in children and adolescents. Primary respiratory arrest seems to be a more common cause than primary cardiac arrest in children 9-13. However, most reports of paediatric cardiac arrest contain insufficient numbers of patients. The main causes of cardiopulmonary arrest in children are congenital malformations, complications of prematurity, sudden infant death syndrome and trauma (NADKARNI et. al, 1998).

The high survival rate of BLS in paediatrics is based on the causes of CPR in children, the possibility of accurate and timely care in the case of early CPR with an emphasis on chest compressions, rapid access to medical services, effective VAS and integrated post-CPR care (GONZALES, 2013).

Despite the knowledge of how important it is for nurses to perform cardiopulmonary resuscitation, theoretical knowledge and scientific papers on VNS and VAS in paediatrics are still incipient. This raises the question: do nurses receive the necessary theoretical training in VNS and VAS in paediatrics?

Answering this question is important because it could help increase knowledge of the current scenario in higher education.

In the face of these accentuations, the nurse's action is the guarantee of life or death (FILGUEIRAS-FILHO, 2013). The decision to study the role of nursing professionals in caring for children in an emergency situation is due to the fact that few studies in the nursing field have focused on this topic and, in this sense, this work is a little explored area.

CHAPTER 2

Objectives

Considering that nursing professionals are usually the first to witness a cardiac arrest in a paediatric hospital, the theoretical knowledge and practical skills of these teams when it comes to BLS and VAS means a greater chance of patient recovery. With this in mind, the aim of this study was to carry out a literature review to analyse the role of nurses and the importance of their theoretical and scientific knowledge in basic and advanced life support in paediatrics.

CHAPTER 3

Materials and Methods

This study follows the pattern of a bibliographical survey, with an integrative review aimed at providing a general illustration of the role of nursing professionals in basic and advanced life support in paediatrics.

The research is classified as bibliographical, as it aims to construct a new form of presentation for a subject that is already known, or even to construct a new theory. The bibliographical review is a resource for this purpose, as it brings together ideas from different sources, synthesising and organising the subject in a more accessible way (FOGLIATTO, 2007).

In turn, Mancini (2007) characterises a literature review as a method that groups together results obtained from research on common subjects, with the aim of synthesising and analysing this data to develop a more comprehensive explanation of a specific phenomenon.

Some authors argue that this methodology has the potential to create a strong knowledge base, capable of guiding professional practice and identifying the need for new research.

The following variables were used to analyse the productions: databases, year of publication; availability of full text and/or abstracts.

After defining the topic, a search was carried out in virtual health databases, the Virtual Health Library (BVS) (http://brasil.bvs.br/), the Virtual Health Library System (LILACS) (http://lilacs.bvsalud.org/), the National Library of Medicine (MEDLINE) (https://www.ncbi.nlm.nih.gov/pubmed/) and the Nursing Database (BDENF) (http://search.bvsalud.org/cvsp/resource/pt/lis-LISBR1.1-17798).

The following descriptors were used: advanced life support in paediatrics, basic life support in paediatrics, cardiac arrest and children. The next step was an exploratory reading of the publications presented in the databases.

The inclusion criteria were: they had been published in the last five years and met the objectives of the study. Those published before 2012 or which did not meet the objectives were excluded.

Considering that the study is based on bibliographical research, there was no need for it to be analysed by the Research Ethics Committee.

Therefore, papers were included because they were related to the theme and objective of this study and met the pre-established inclusion criteria.

The scarcity of materials available on the subject made the search difficult, generating a small number of studies. To further support the discussion, dissertations and theses on the subject were used.

CHAPTER 4

Results and Discussion

Taking into account all the criteria for inclusion and exclusion of articles, as well as the use of descriptors, 26 articles published between 2012 and 2017 were found. However, in order to achieve the aim of this study, only the 10 publications found in the International Health Sciences Literature (MEDLINE) will be used. When analysing the distribution of articles by database, it was found that of the 26 articles, 10 (39%) were found in the International Health Sciences Literature (MEDLINE), 4 (15%) were found in the Virtual Health Library (BVS) database, 5 (19%) were found in the Virtual Health Library System (LILACS) and finally 7 (27%) articles were found in the Nursing Database (BDENF), as can be seen in Table 1. This result shows that few articles on the subject are being produced and published in scientific journals.

TABLE 1: Distribution of articles by database.

Database	N	%
Virtual Health Library BBVS	4	15
Virtual Health Library System - *LILACS*	5	19
National Library of Medicine - MELHNEE	10	39
Nursing Databases BBDEFF	7	27

Matsumo (2012a) presents a review of the epidemiology, causes, diagnosis and management of cardiac arrest in children. Her work shows that, unlike in adults, sudden cardiac arrest in children is rare, and that when it does occur, it is usually caused by respiratory failure and/or shock. In this context, early recognition and immediate treatment of these conditions can prevent cardiac arrest and improve the outcome of these patients.

This is why paediatric assessment is important in emergency situations, as it enables rapid and efficient recognition of signs of respiratory failure and/or shock. This recognition allows patients to be treated in these situations, which makes it possible to prevent cardiopulmonary failure and cardiac arrest in children (MATSUNO 2012b).

Continuous training for nurses should be encouraged when it comes to CPR care.

Since most of the nurses who took part in the study were unaware of some of the procedures recommended by current cardiopulmonary resuscitation guidelines, as well as the ideal sequence of care. Since nurses are usually the first professionals to encounter patients in cardiopulmonary resuscitation (CPR), continuing education will help restore the life process and provide effective patient care. In this context, it is recommended that health services carry out periodic training in CPR in order to train teams, especially nurses, to provide fast, safe and effective care, in accordance with the recommendations, and to maintain homogeneity of behaviour among teams (ALVES et. al, 2013).

Thinking about the role of nurses in basic life support, the question arises as to how this is done in the case of paediatric urgencies and emergencies. In their study, GIURIATTI et. al (2014) proposed standardising nursing intervention in the face of paediatric cardiopulmonary arrest and also proposed that the hospital should draw up a document in which all the operational procedures are recorded, thus forming a CPR Technical Standard to guide nursing care, qualifying the service so that it can be used in other hospitals, since there is a shortage of material on the subject and there is a complexity to CPR that calls for standardisation and training of all the teams in an interdisciplinary way to act in an organised and harmonious manner, with good leadership as well as good leadership, harmonious manner, with good leadership, as well as acting in an agile and precise manner to achieve success in CPR.

This is important because it was found that there is no protocol to guide the team in cases of CPR, as they reported acting in a heterogeneous manner. In addition, there was insufficient knowledge of current protocols, as well as unpreparedness to carry out certain procedures, primary assessment and chest compressions in accordance with the guidelines proposed by the American Heart Association, which can be a hindrance to the quality of care provided to children and adults (ABRANTES et. al, 2015).

Among other aspects that make it difficult to provide care during a CPR, performance in carrying out correct care is crucial, and this is provided by various factors that directly influence the desired result. Notably, the aspect related to knowledge is always present in this and the studies cited, but an interesting feature of this study is the identification of difficulties in the work process and in the ambience or physical structure. It was found that professionals are able to identify the occurrence of a CA, however it seems essential to train the team to act in extreme emergency conditions (MORAES et. al, 2016).

A study assessed the knowledge of the nursing team in relation to the Cardiopulmonary Resuscitation technique and the medications used in children admitted to the Paediatric Intensive Care Unit of the General Hospital of Vitória da Conquista, Bahia. The results of this research showed that of the 25 nursing professionals in the Paediatric Intensive Care Unit studied, 20% were trained after admission and 36% received no training, having to learn the service on a daily basis while carrying out their duties. The team surveyed was able to successfully recognise respiratory failure in children, but when trying to identify cardiopulmonary arrest they were unable to demonstrate their technical-scientific knowledge satisfactorily, as they gave incomplete answers relating to all the signs and symptoms of its onset. The research points out that an important point to be worked on for the staff in question would be the use of drugs, focussing on the cause/effect on the organism of the child with cardiopulmonary arrest (SANTOS, 2017).

This field is difficult to study, mainly due to the low level of participation in the questionnaires and the small sample size, which prevent the findings from being generalised. Based on the results, it is possible to infer that the New CPR Guidelines, launched in October 2010, have not been implemented in practice, and that permanent education interventions are needed for the paediatric emergency healthcare team to ensure effective CPR (BERTOLO et. al, 2014).

The care of critically ill paediatric patients can take place in a variety of settings, whether pre- or in-hospital. This is why the training of the care team must be sought. This training, which can take the form of courses accredited by organisations and associations, is fundamental to improving the quality of care. It is recommended that all doctors and nurses, especially those who work with critically ill patients, take the Paediatric Advanced Life Support (PALS) course and recertify every two years (PESSOA, et. al, 2016).

There are countless challenges to be overcome in nursing care for children in the emergency network, and this care is of great importance for improving their clinical condition. It is necessary to have trained professionals who are able to meet the demand in the emergency network, carrying out specific procedures based on humanised and appropriate care for the child. There is a noticeable lack of specific nursing studies in the area of nursing care in paediatric emergencies, which is an important area of care. Finally, it is understood that more research should be carried out on this subject due to its relevance not only to nursing professionals but also to society (ANDRADE et. al, 2017).

CHAPTER 5

Final considerations

The aim of this study was to find out how nurses work and the importance of their knowledge of basic and advanced life support in paediatrics for successful resuscitation of children.

After analysing the studies, it was possible to conclude that there are few studies on this subject, and that the knowledge of the nursing team in this regard is still incipient. This study made it possible to identify the importance of nurses' theoretical and scientific knowledge within institutions that care for children at risk of cardiac arrest. This knowledge enables them to provide more agile care by organising the team based on their theoretical background. The nurses in the units combine theoretical background (essential) with leadership skills, perceptive work, initiative, teaching skills, maturity and emotional stability.

We therefore realise the need to invest in training for the professionals who provide direct assistance to patients in cardiac arrest.

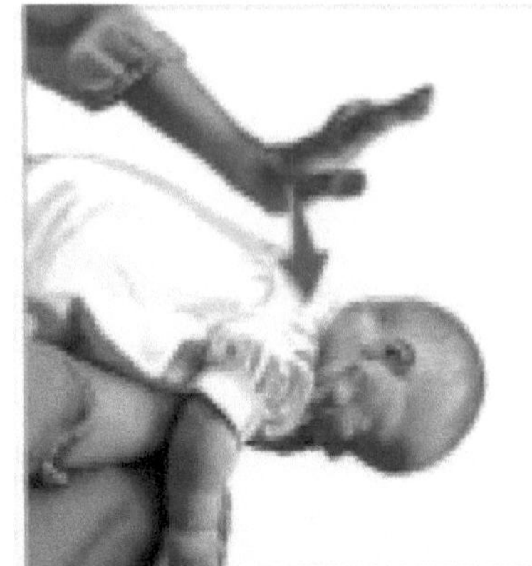
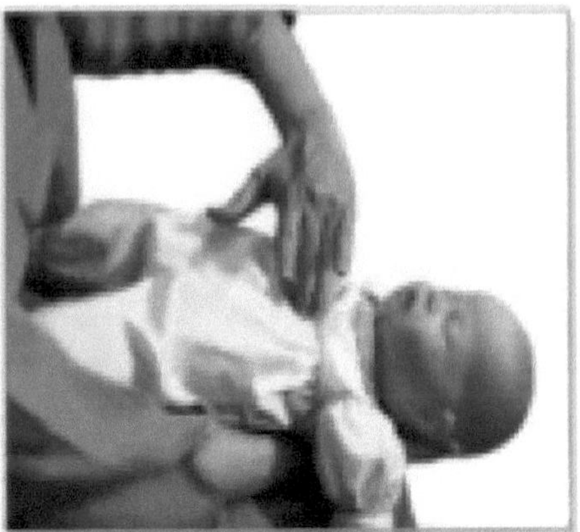
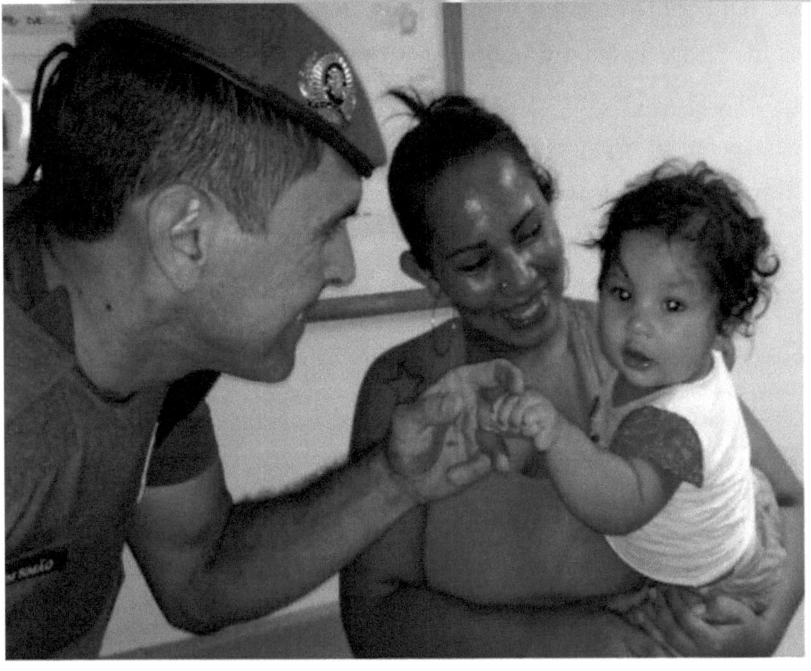

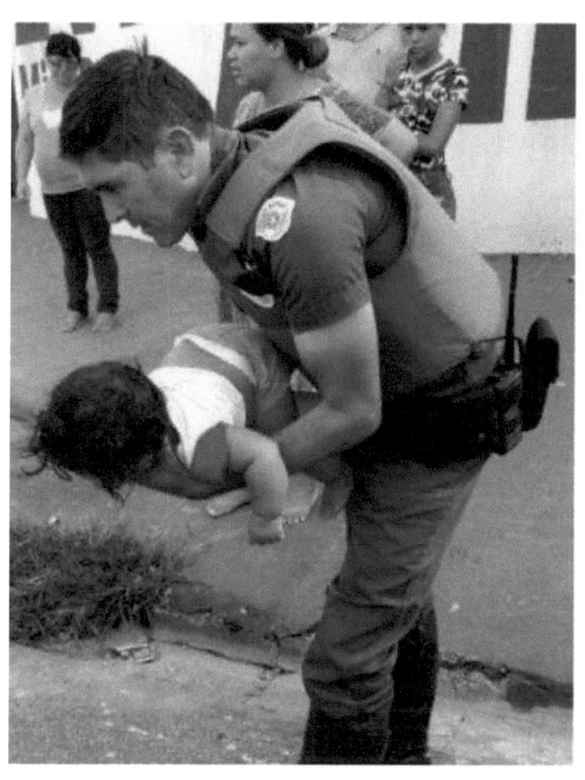

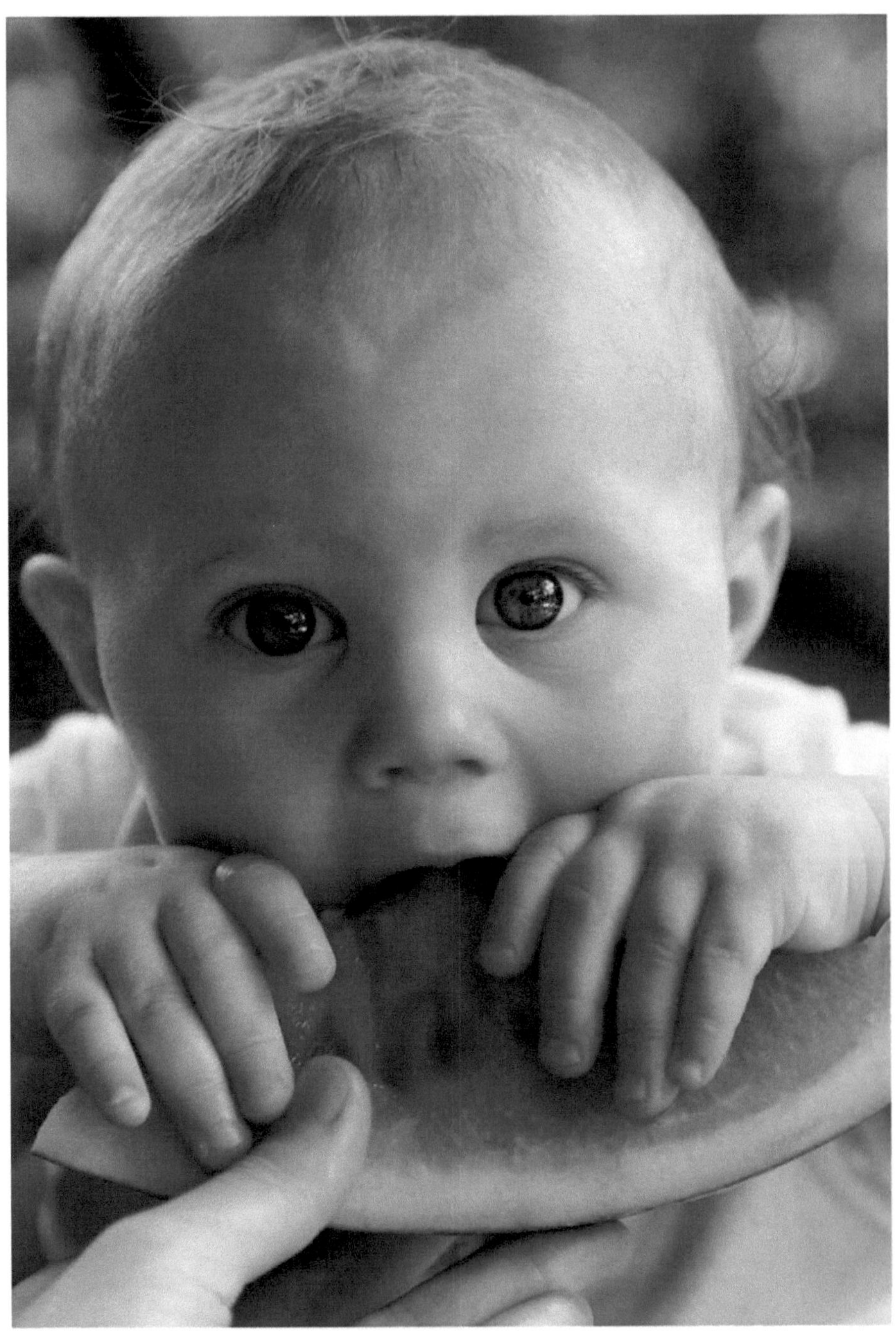

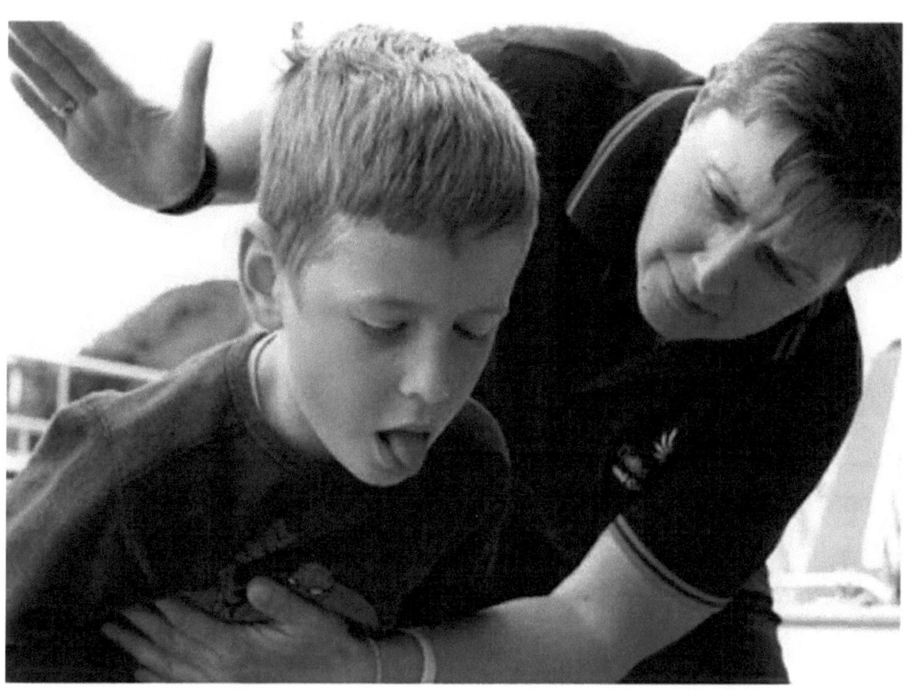

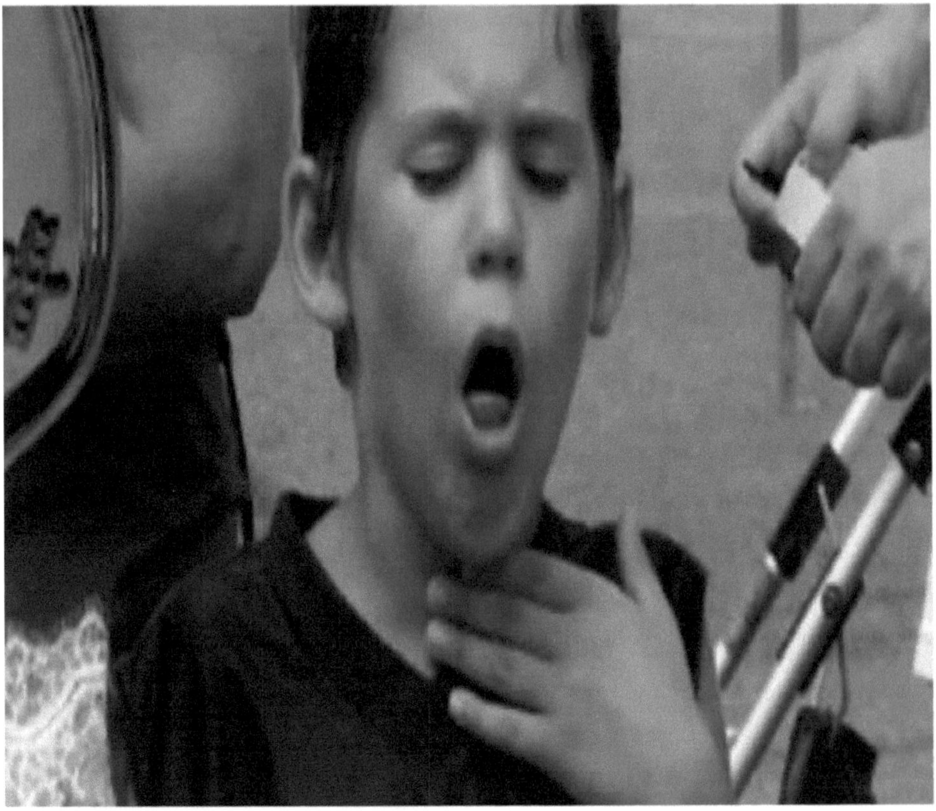

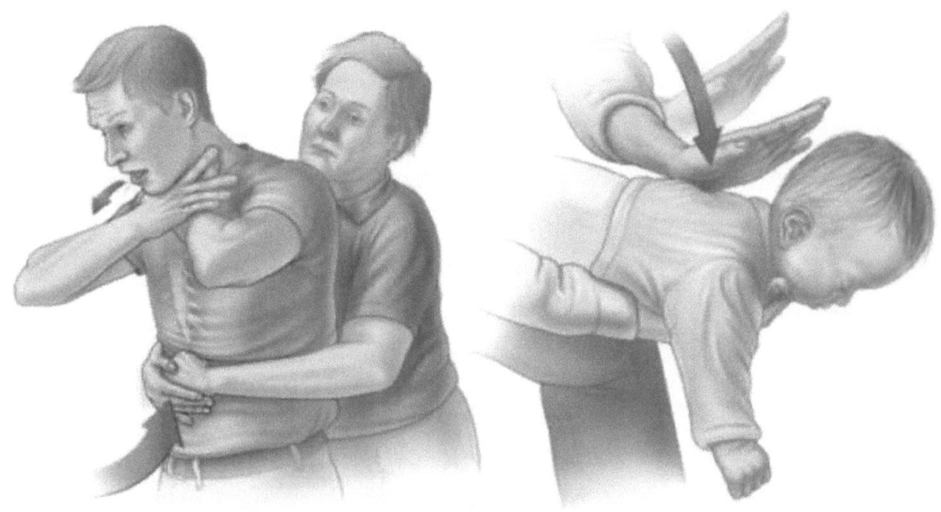

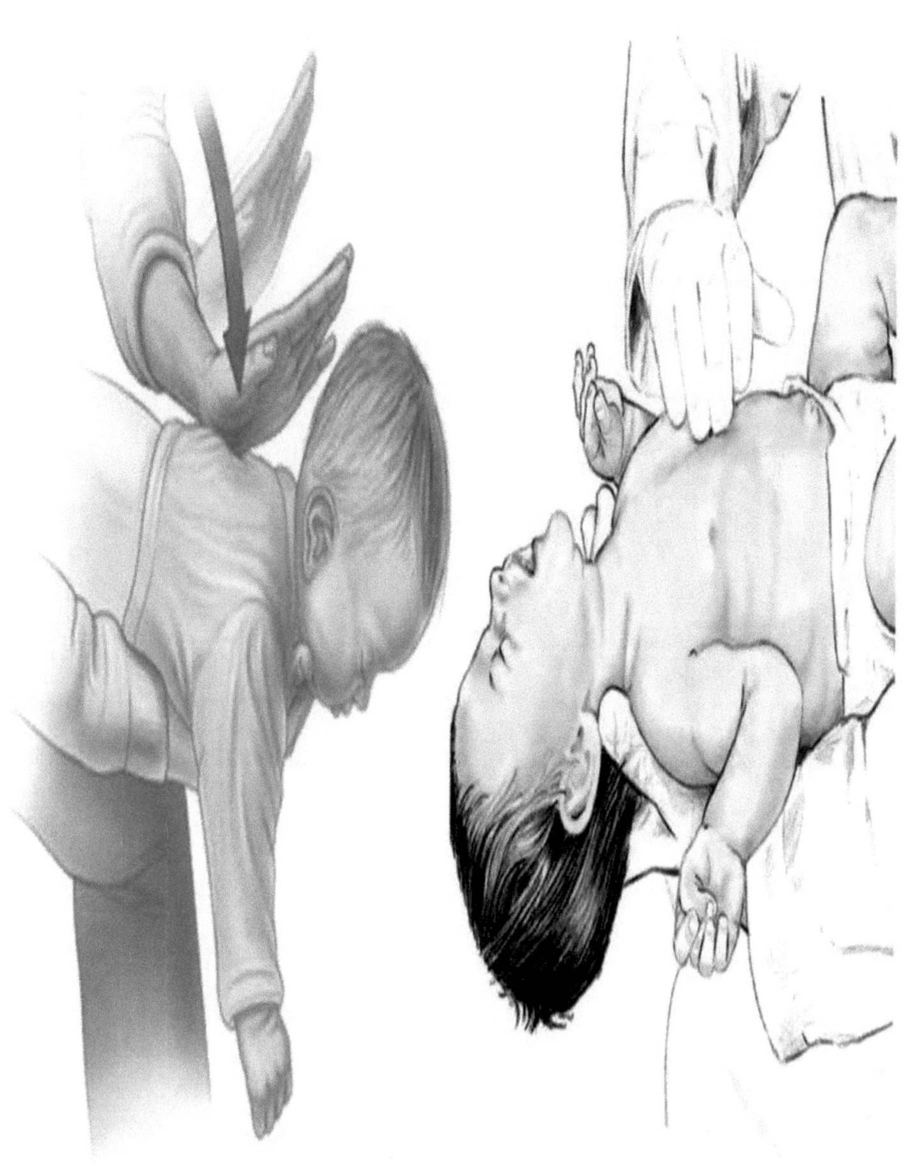

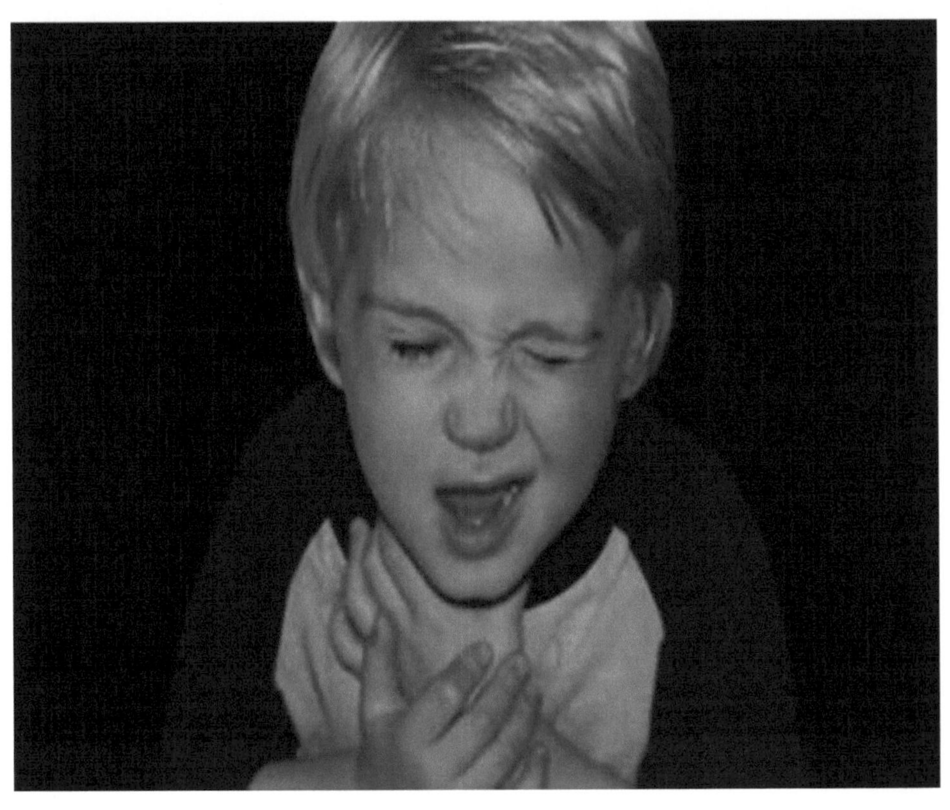

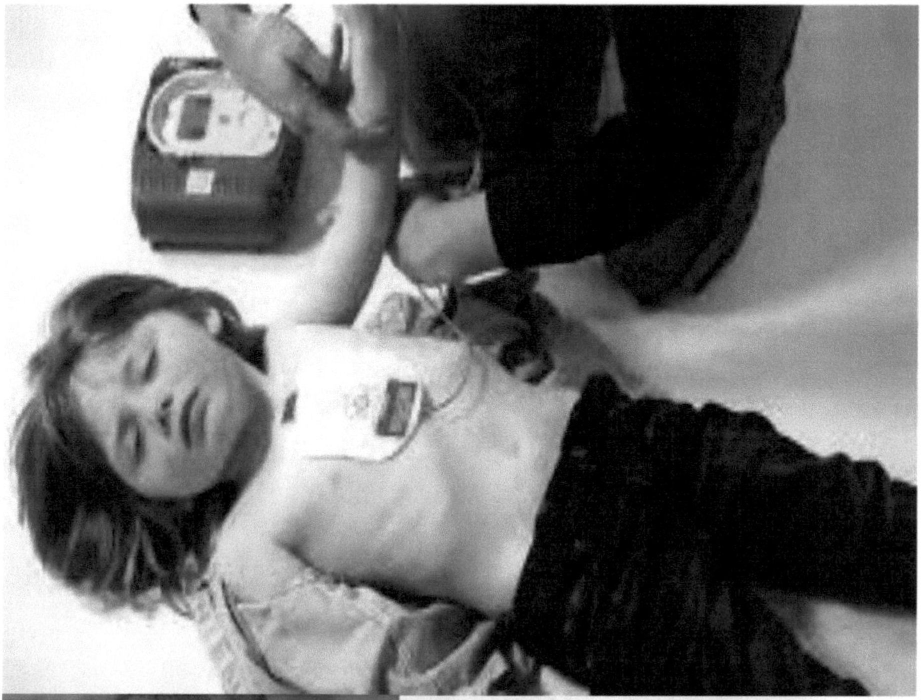

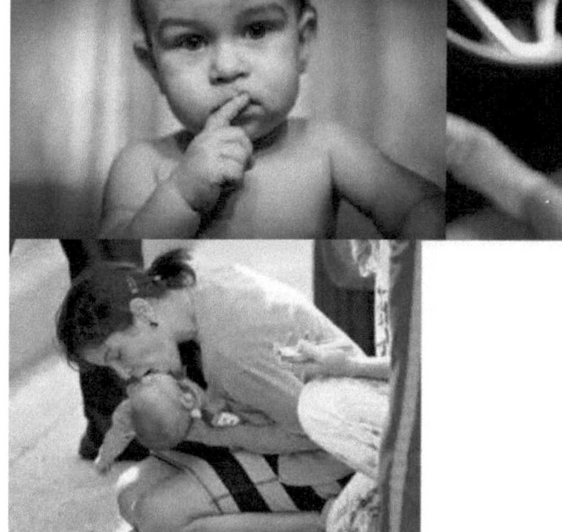

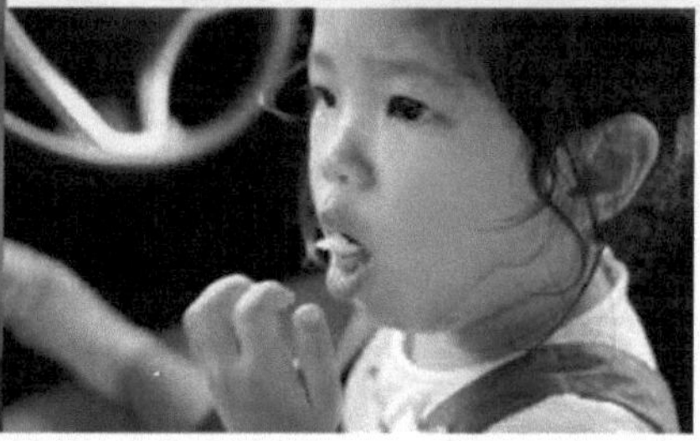

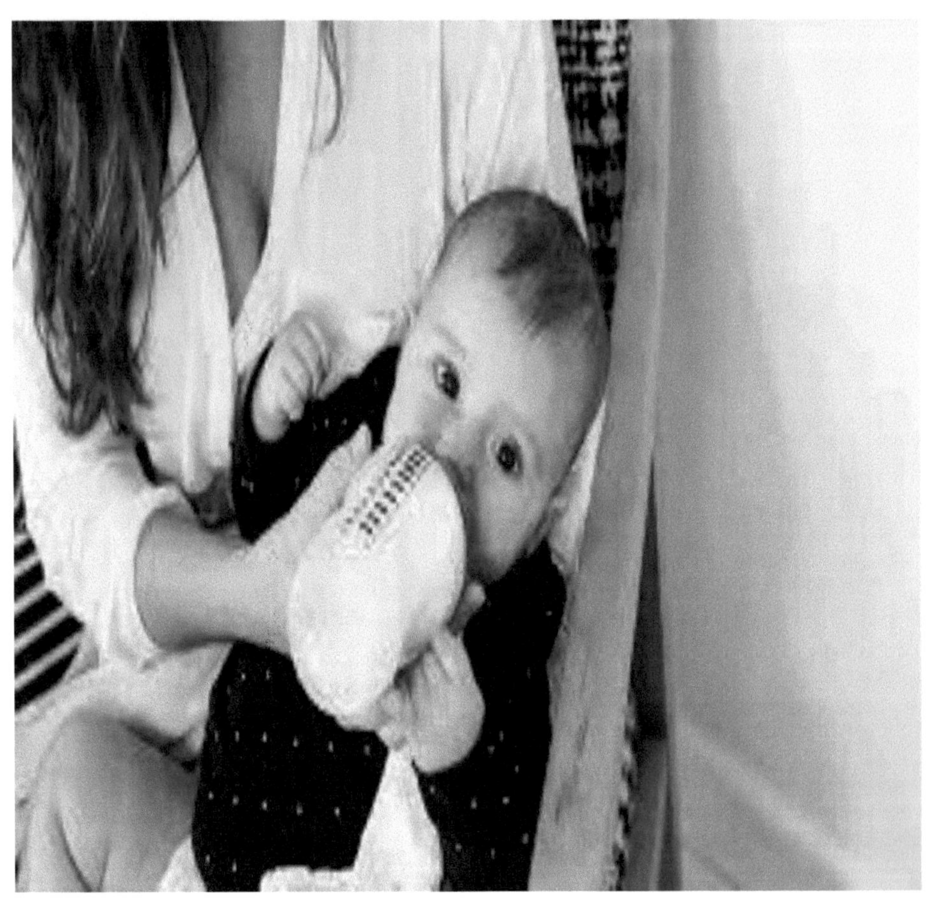

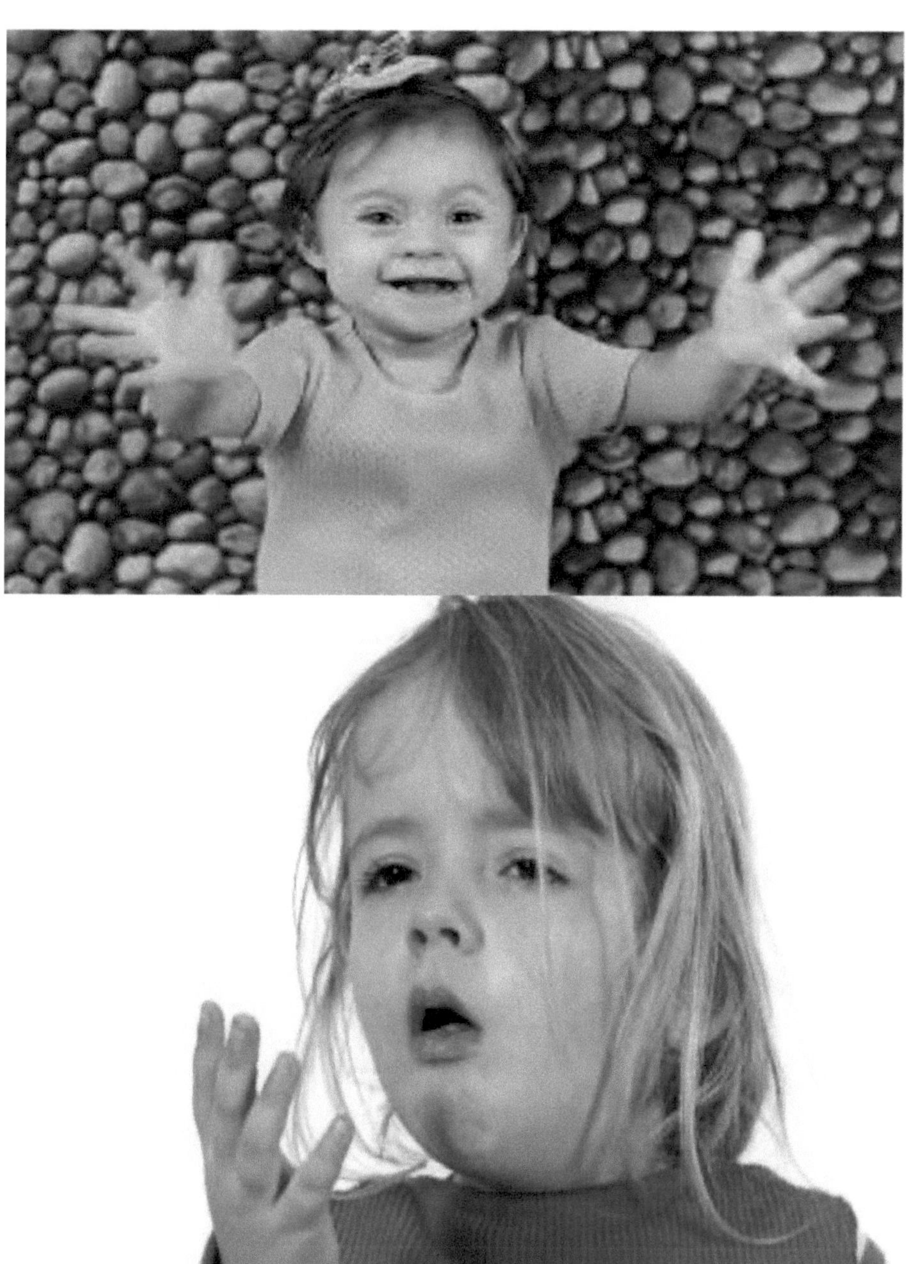

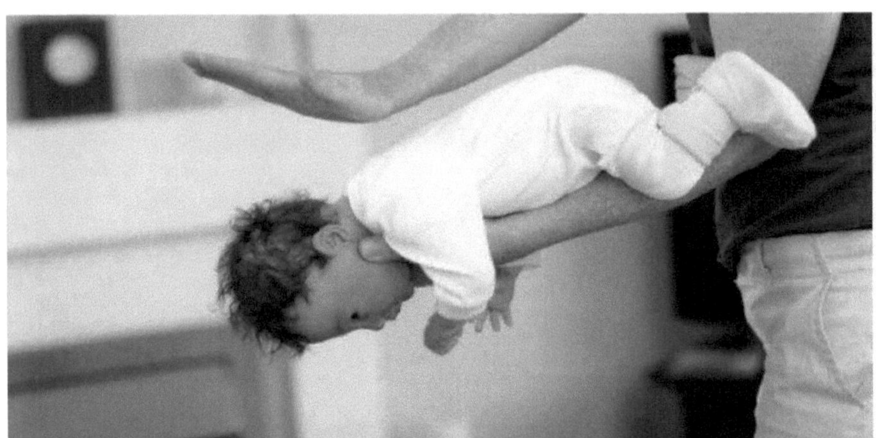

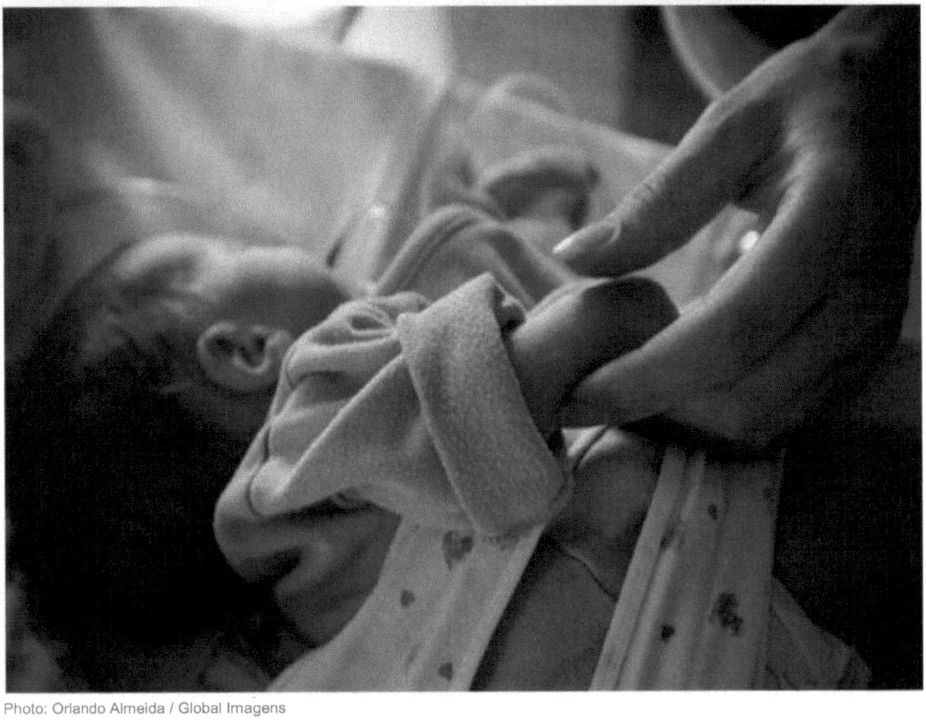

Photo: Orlando Almeida / Global Imagens

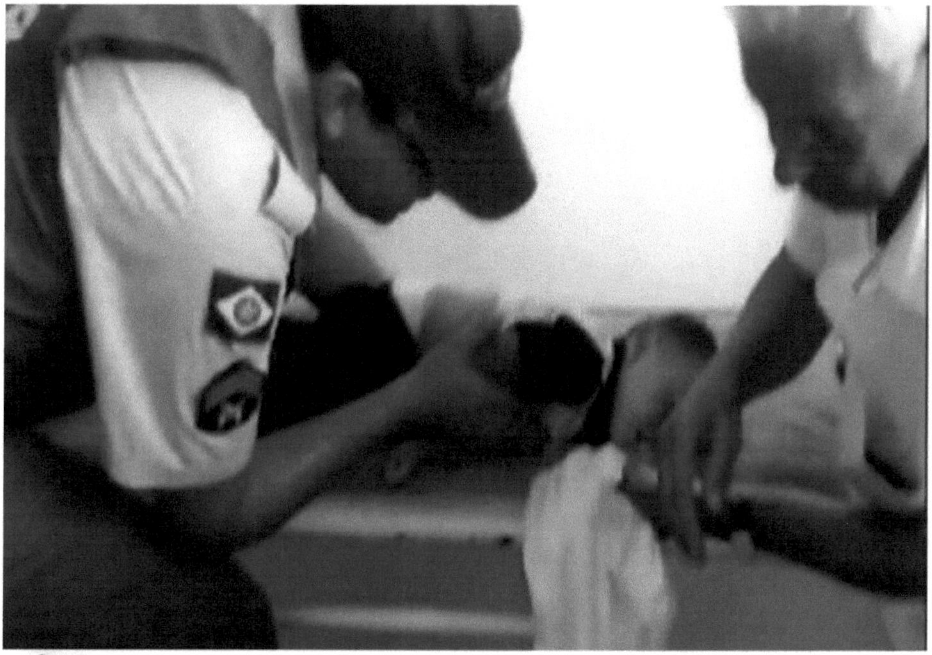

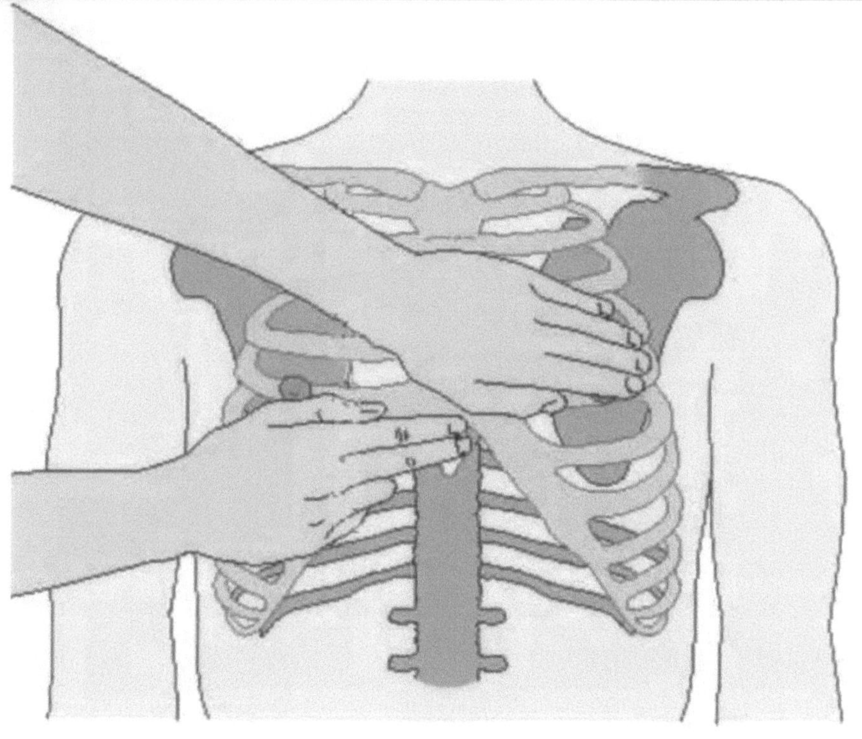

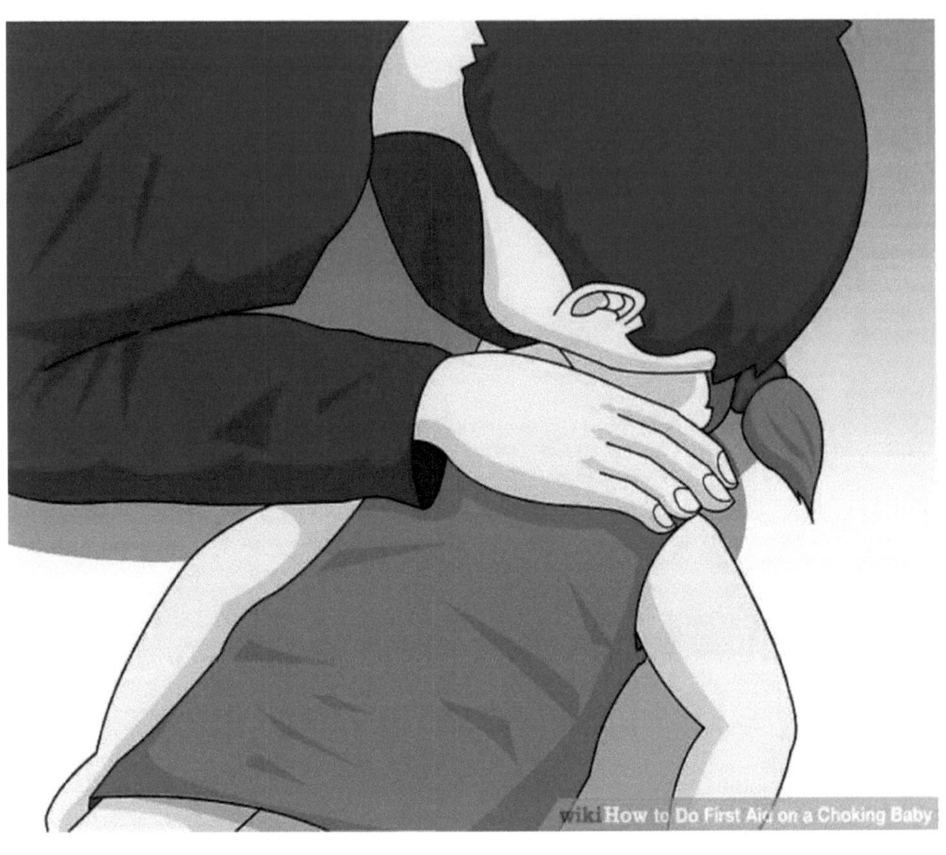
wikiHow to Do First Aid on a Choking Baby

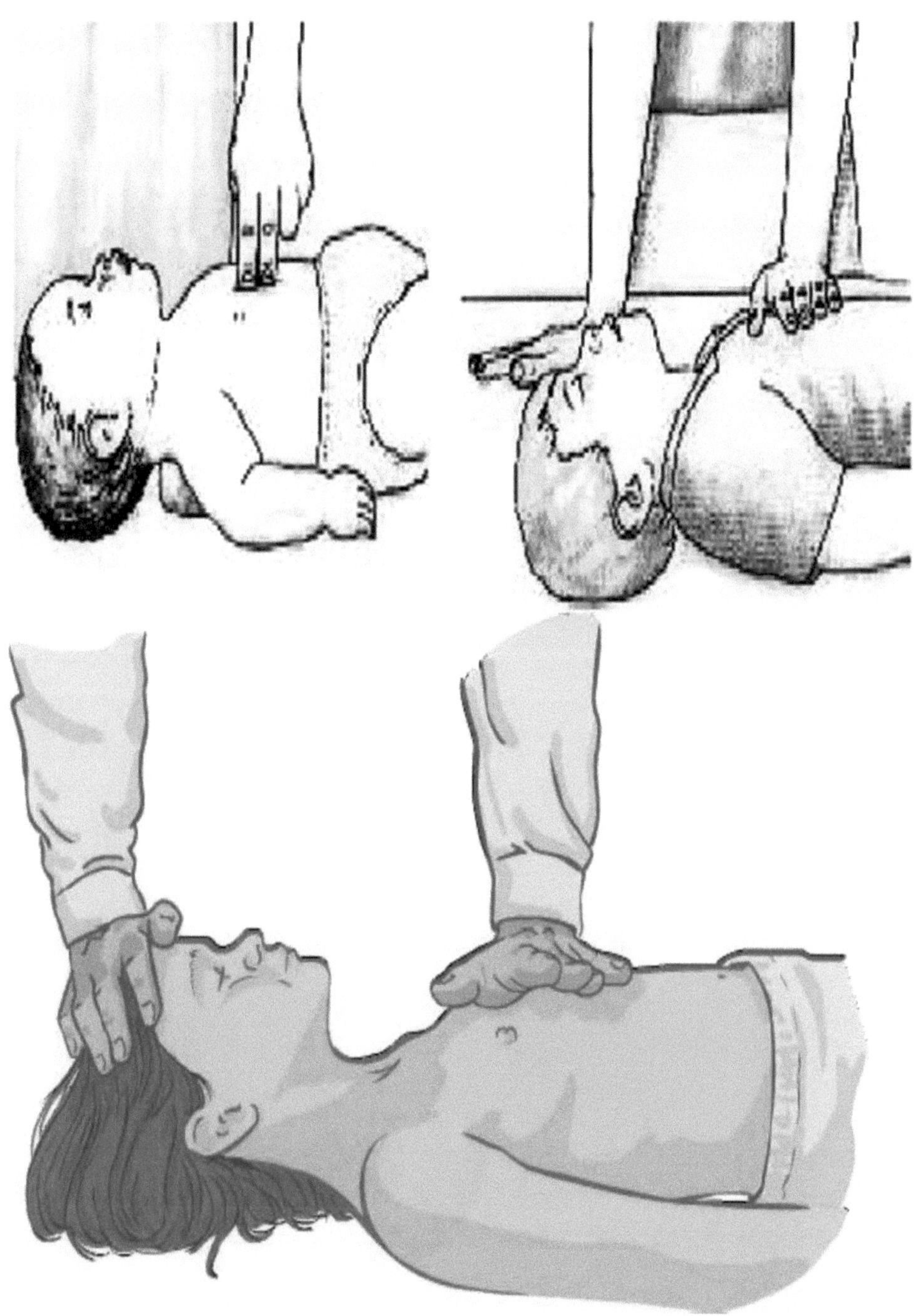

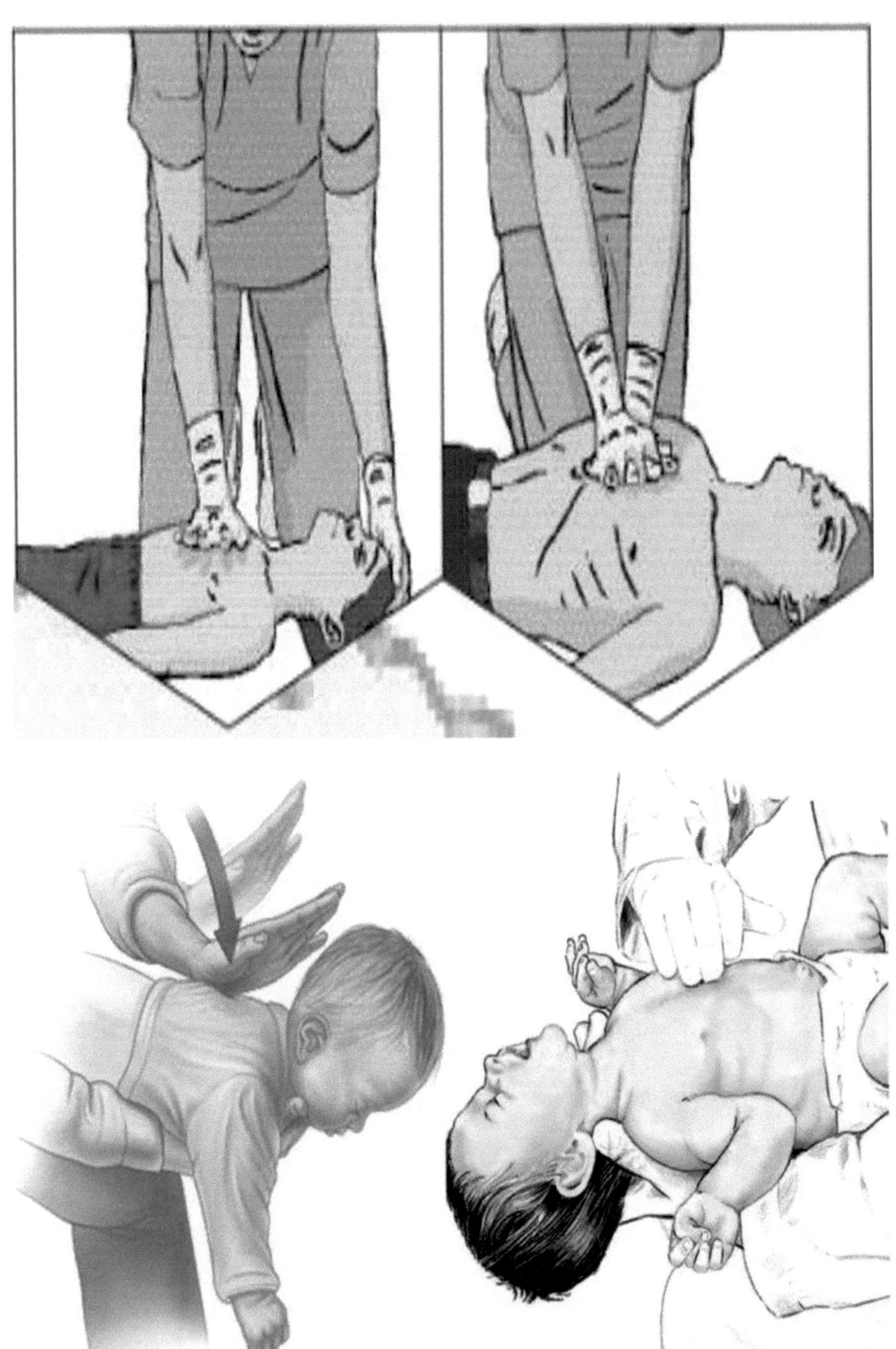

Placenta Normal al Flujo Sanguíneo Cerebral

Cerebro

La flecha indica flujo de sangre rica normal

Corazón

Placenta

Cordón umbilical

Disminución del Flujo Sanguíneo al Cerebro

Disminución del suministro de sangre conduce a un estado de isquemia. Células cerebrales mueren sin flujo sanguíneo adecuado y oxígeno.

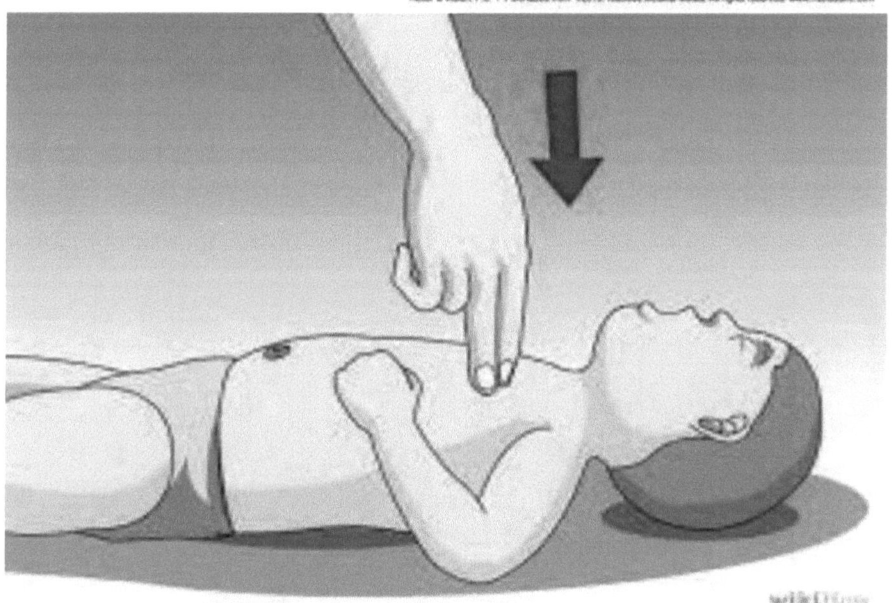

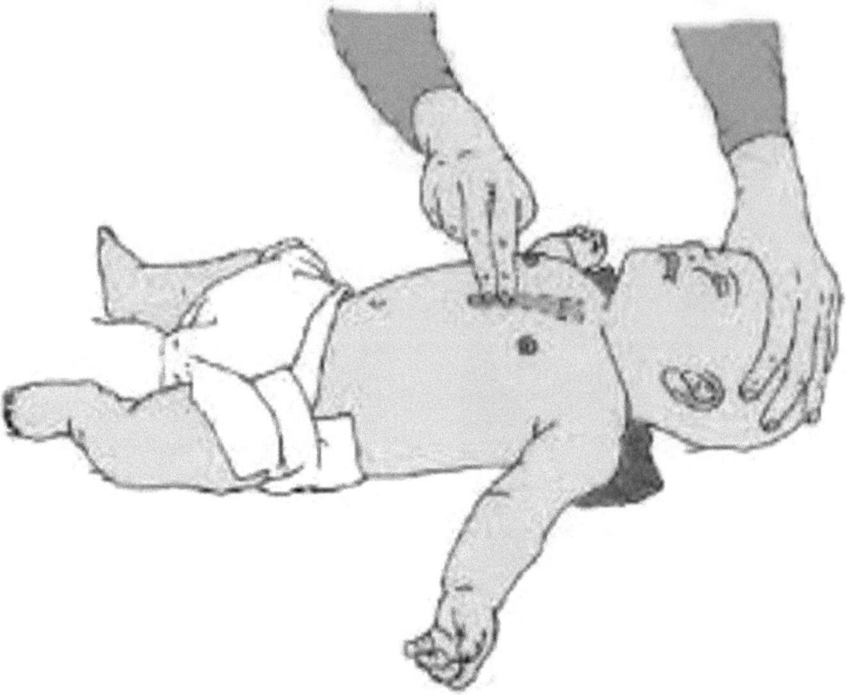

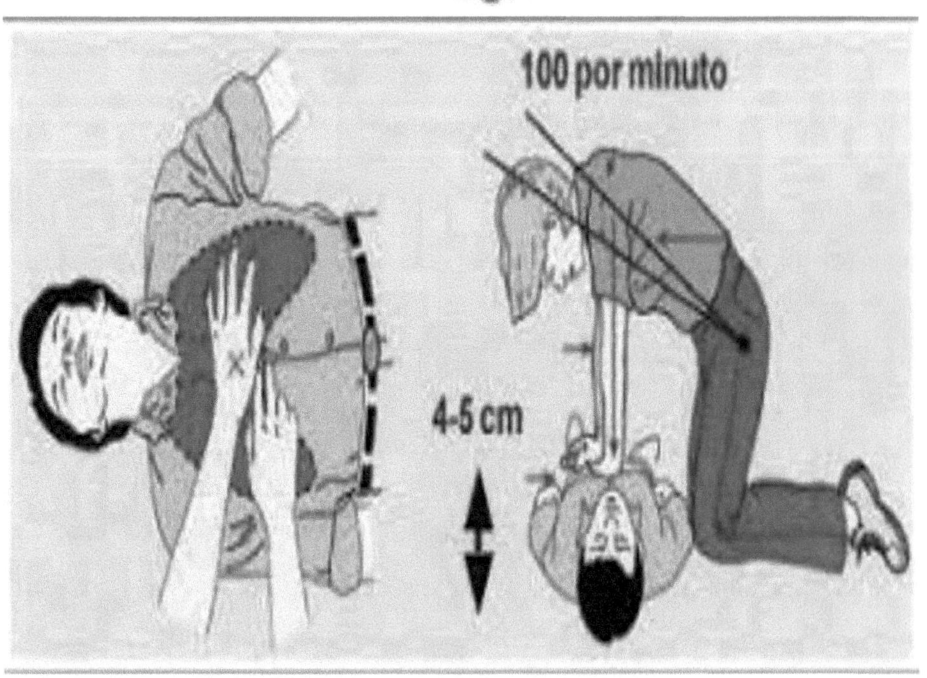
100 por minuto
4-5 cm

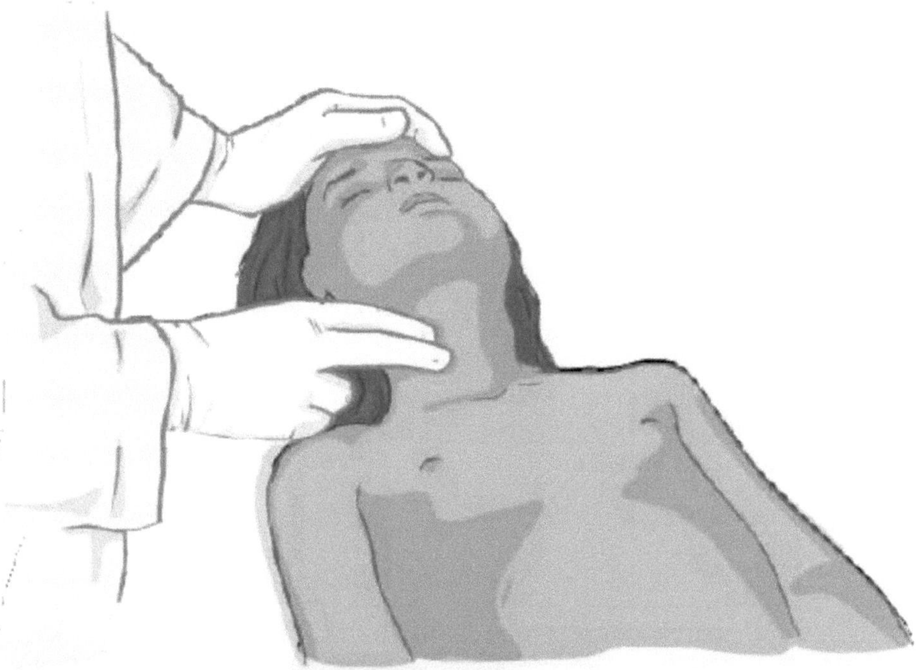

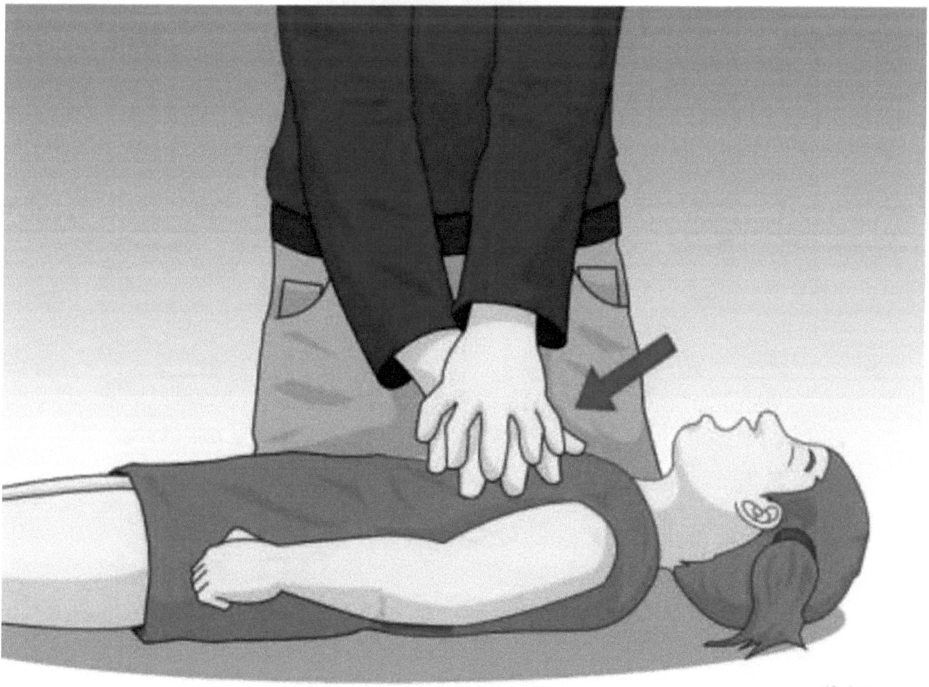

wikiHow

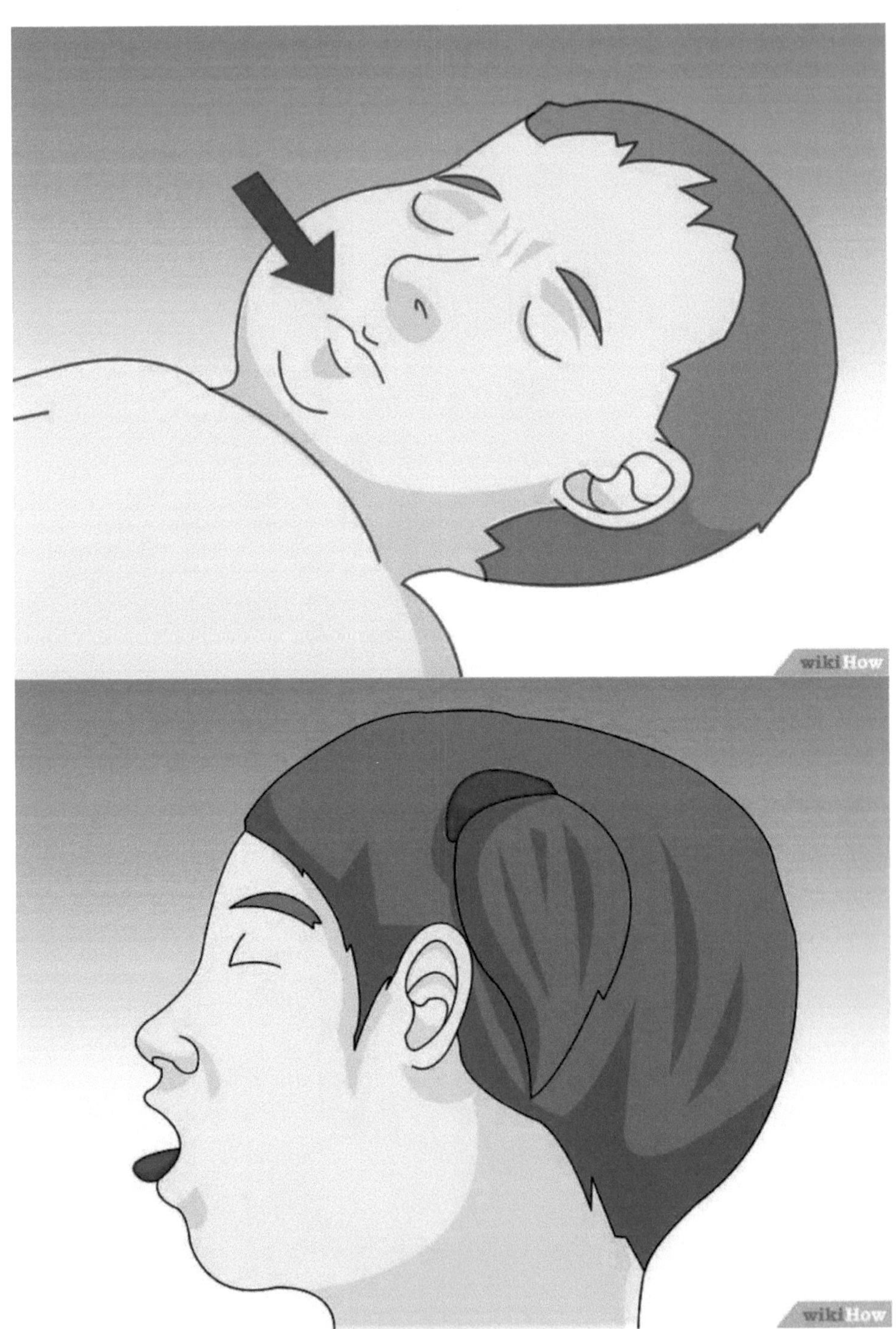
wikiHow
wikiHow

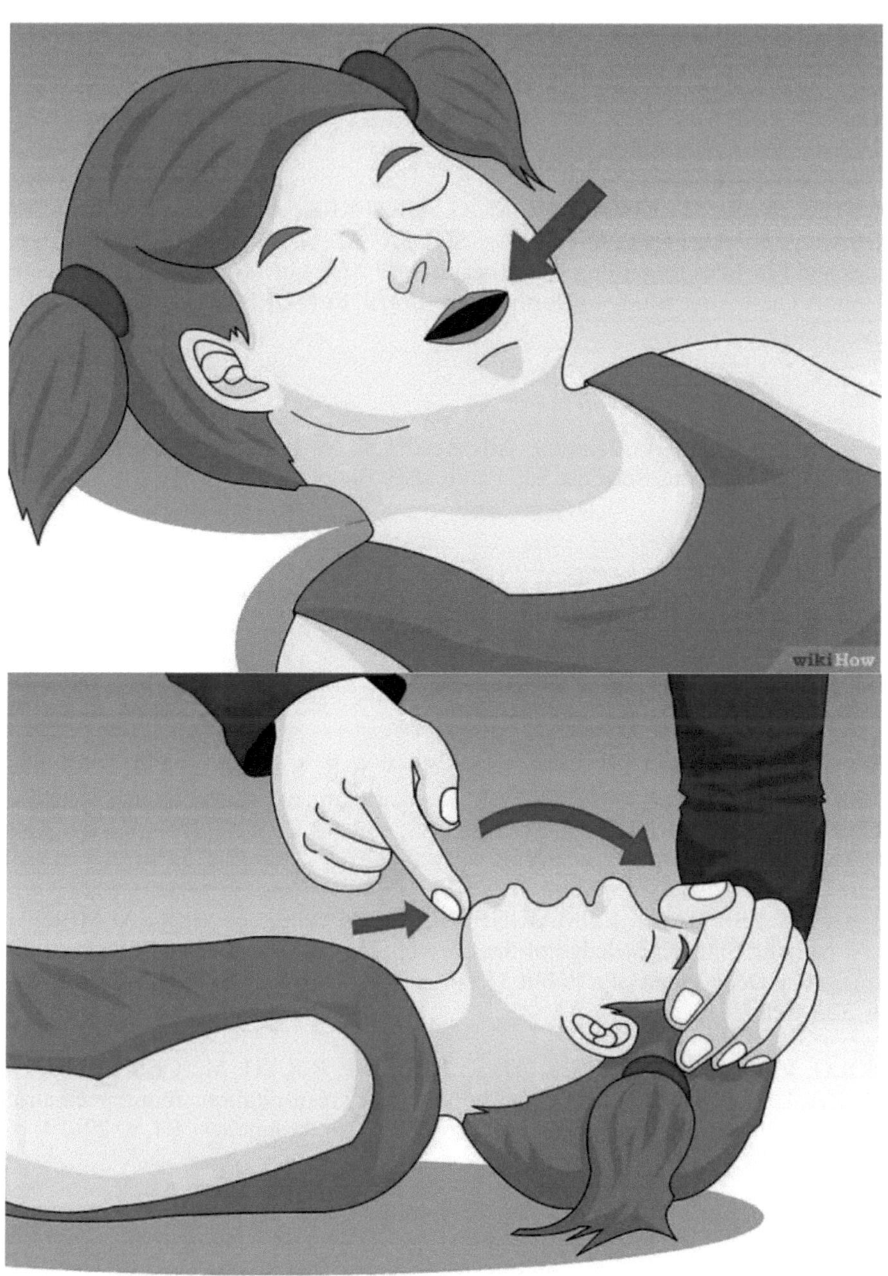
wikiHow

CHAPTER 6

References

ABRANTES, A. W. B.; COURA, E. M. G.; BEZERRA, A. L. D.; ASSIS, E. V.; FEITOSA, A. N. A.; FREITAS, M. A.; SOUSA, M. N. A. Nursing Knowledge, Attitudes and Practices Regarding Cardiorespiratory Arrest in a Neonatal Intermediate Care Unit: A Qualitative Study in Northeastern Brazil. Rev. ORIGINAL RESEARCH, n. 25, v. 1, 2015.

AHA - American Heart Association. Advanced Life Support in Paediatrics, health professional's book. Prous Science, São Paulo - SP, Brazil, 2008.

ALVES, C. A.; BARBOSA, C. N. S.; FARIA, H. T. G. Cardiorespiratory arrest and nursing: Knowledge about basic life support. Rev. Cogitare Enferm. n. 18, v. 2, p. 296-301, 2013.

ANDRADE, A. K. M.; MATOS, M. L. S.; SILVA, R. S.; GALLOTTI, F. C. M.; OLIVEIRA, C. G. S. Nurse performance in paediatric urgent and emergency services. In: INTERNATIONAL NURSING CONGRESS, p. 9- 12, 2017.

ARAÚJO, L. P.; SILVA, A. L.; MARINELLI, N. P.; POSSO, M. B. S.; ALMEIDA, L. M. N. Nursing Staff Knowledge of the Cardiopulmonary Resuscitation Protocol in the Emergency Department of a Public Hospital. Rev. Univap, São José dos Campos-SP, , n. 32, v. 18, 2012.

BERTOLO, V. F.; RODRIGUES, C. D. S.; RIBEIRO, R. C. H. M.; CESARINO, C. B.; SOUZA, L. H; Knowledge about cardiopulmonary resuscitation among paediatric emergency health professionals. Rev enferm UERJ, Rio de Janeiro - RJ, n. 22v. 4, p. 54650, 2014.

FERREIRA, A. V. S. Basic Life Support. Rev Soc *Cardiol. São* Paulo - SP, n. 11, v. 2, p. 214 - 225, 2001.

FILGUEIRAS - FILHO, N. M.; BANDEIRA, A. C.; DELMONDES, T,; OLIVEIRA, A.; LIMA, J. R. A. S,; CRUZ, V. Evaluation of the general knowledge of emergency physicians from hospitals in Salvador, Bahia, about the care of victims with arrest. cardiorespiratory. *Rev. Arq Bras Cardiol.* n. 87, p. 634-40, 2006.

FOGLIATTO, F. Organisation of Scientific Texts , 2007. Available at:<http://www.producao.ufrgs.br/arquivos/disciplinas/146_seminario_de_pesquisa_2_dir etrizes_referencial_teorico.doc.>. Accessed on: 25 September 2017.

GIURIATTI, M. P. Z. A.; ASCARI, R. A.; FERRAZ, L.; NEISS, M. Technical Standard for Nursing Intervention in Paediatric Cardiorespiratory Arrest. *Rev. Brazilian Journal of Surgery and Clinical Research.* v.6, n. 2, p.11-17, mar - mai, 2014.

GOMBOTZ, H.; WEH, B.; MITTERNDORFER, W.; REHAK, P. In-hospital cardiac resuscitation outside the ICU by nursing staff equipped with automated external defibrillators - the first 500 cases. *Rev. Resuscitation.* n. 70, v. 3, 70 p. 416-22, 2006.

GUSSON, A. C. T.; LOPES, J. C. Paediatrics in the 21st century: a speciality in danger. *Rev Paul Pediatr*, n. 28, v. 1, p. 115-20, 2010.

HORSTED, T.; RASMUSSEN, L. S.; MEYHOFF, C. S.; NIELSEN, S. L. Long-term prognosis after out-ofhospital cardiac arrest. *Rev. Resuscitation.* n. 72, v. 1, p. 214-218, 2007.

LIMA, S. G.; MACEDO, L. A.; VIDAL, M. D. E. L.; SÁ, M. P. Continuing Education in BLS and CVAS: Impact on the Knowledge of Nursing Professionals. Rev. Arq Bras Cardiol. n, 93, p. 582-588, 2009.

MANCINI, M.C. Systematic review studies: a guide to carefully synthesising scientific evidence, 2007. Available at:<http://www.scielo.br/pdf/rbfis/v11n1/12.pdf.>. Accessed on: 25 September 2017.

MATSUMO, A. K. Cardiac arrest in children. *Rev. Medicina,* São Paulo - SP, n. 45, p. 223-33, 2012.

MORAES, C. L. K.; PAULA, G. M. A.; SILVA, J. R.; RODRIGUES, M. C. L. Challenges Faced by the Nursing Team in Cardiopulmonary Resuscitation in a Hospital Emergency Unit Rev. Eletrônica Estácio Saúde, n. 1, v. 5, 2016.

MOULE, P.; ALBARRAN, J. W.; Automated external defibrillation as part BLS: implications for education and practice. Rev. Resuscitation. n. 54, v. 3, p. 223-30, 2002.

NADKARNI, V.; HAZINSKI, M. F.; ZIDEMAN, D.; KATTWINKEL, J.; QUAN, L.; BINGHAM, R.; ZARITTSKY, A.; BLAND, J.; KRAMER, E.; TIBALLS, J. LIFE SUPPORT IN PAEDIATRICS. A Statement of the Recommendations of the Paediatric Life Support Working Group of the International Liaison Resuscitation Committee. Rev. Arq Bras Cardiol. n. 5, v. 70, 1998.

PESSOA, F. M.; FERREIRA, .A. R.; MELO, M. C. B.; GRESTA, M. M.; VASCONCELLOS, M. C. Basic and advanced life support in paediatrics: history of implementation in Minas Gerais and update. Rev Med Minas Gerais, n. 26, 2016.

TACSI, Y. R. C VENDRUSCOLO DMS. Nursing assistance in paediatric emergency services. Rev. Latino-Am. Enfermagem. 2004;12(3):477-84.

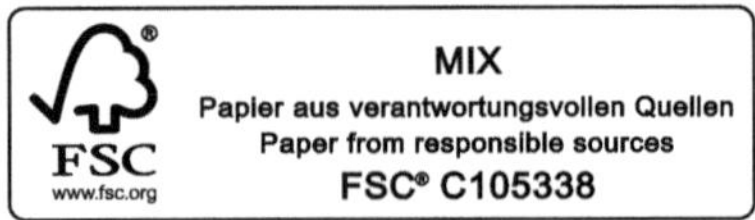

Printed by Books on Demand GmbH, Norderstedt / Germany